Name Juliana –

Contact No

E-mail

Address

Blood Group   Age

Doctor's Name

Doctor's No

Pharmacy Name

Pharmacy No

EMERGENCY CONTACTS

Name Caitlin Armstrong

Contact No 216·410·6287

Name

Contact No

Name

Contact No

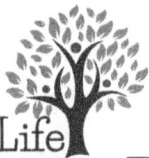

NOTES

NOTES

Week : 3·25 - 3·31				Weight :	
Date	Meal	Time	Before	After	Med/Insulin
MON	Breakfast				
	Lunch				
	Dinner				
	Bedtime				

Notes :

Date	Meal	Time	Before	After	Med/Insulin
TUE	Breakfast	1157	194		5 units
	Lunch				
	Dinner	10:19	255		8.5
	Bedtime	9:47	187		Ø

Notes :

Date	Meal	Time	Before	After	Med/Insulin
WED	Breakfast		258		
	Lunch				
	Dinner				
	Bedtime				

Notes :

Date	Meal	Time	Before	After	Med/Insulin
THU	Breakfast				
	Lunch				
	Dinner				
	Bedtime				

Notes :

Date	Meal	Time	Before	After	Med/Insulin
FRI	Breakfast				
	Lunch				
	Dinner				
	Bedtime				

Notes :

Date	Meal	Time	Before	After	Med/Insulin
SAT	Breakfast				
	Lunch				
	Dinner				
	Bedtime				

Notes :

Date	Meal	Time	Before	After	Med/Insulin
SUN	Breakfast				
	Lunch				
	Dinner				
	Bedtime				

Notes :

Notes :

Week :					Weight :

Date	Meal	Time	Before	After	Med/Insulin
MON	Breakfast				
	Lunch				
	Dinner				
	Bedtime				

Notes :

Date	Meal	Time	Before	After	Med/Insulin
TUE	Breakfast				
	Lunch				
	Dinner				
	Bedtime				

Notes :

Date	Meal	Time	Before	After	Med/Insulin
WED	Breakfast				
	Lunch				
	Dinner				
	Bedtime				

Notes :

Date	Meal	Time	Before	After	Med/Insulin
THU	Breakfast				
	Lunch				
	Dinner				
	Bedtime				

Notes :

Date	Meal	Time	Before	After	Med/Insulin
FRI	Breakfast				
	Lunch				
	Dinner				
	Bedtime				

Notes :

Date	Meal	Time	Before	After	Med/Insulin
SAT	Breakfast				
	Lunch				
	Dinner				
	Bedtime				

Notes :

Date	Meal	Time	Before	After	Med/Insulin
SUN	Breakfast				
	Lunch				
	Dinner				
	Bedtime				

Notes :

Notes :

Week :				Weight :	
Date	Meal	Time	Before	After	Med/Insulin
MON	Breakfast				
	Lunch				
	Dinner				
	Bedtime				

Notes :

Date	Meal	Time	Before	After	Med/Insulin
TUE	Breakfast				
	Lunch				
	Dinner				
	Bedtime				

Notes :

Date	Meal	Time	Before	After	Med/Insulin
WED	Breakfast				
	Lunch				
	Dinner				
	Bedtime				

Notes :

Date	Meal	Time	Before	After	Med/Insulin
THU	Breakfast				
	Lunch				
	Dinner				
	Bedtime				

Notes :

Date	Meal	Time	Before	After	Med/Insulin
FRI	Breakfast				
	Lunch				
	Dinner				
	Bedtime				

Notes :

Date	Meal	Time	Before	After	Med/Insulin
SAT	Breakfast				
	Lunch				
	Dinner				
	Bedtime				

Notes :

Date	Meal	Time	Before	After	Med/Insulin
SUN	Breakfast				
	Lunch				
	Dinner				
	Bedtime				

Notes :

Notes :

Week :				Weight :	
Date	**Meal**	**Time**	**Before**	**After**	**Med/Insulin**
MON	Breakfast				
	Lunch				
	Dinner				
	Bedtime				
Notes :					
Date	**Meal**	**Time**	**Before**	**After**	**Med/Insulin**
TUE	Breakfast				
	Lunch				
	Dinner				
	Bedtime				
Notes :					
Date	**Meal**	**Time**	**Before**	**After**	**Med/Insulin**
WED	Breakfast				
	Lunch				
	Dinner				
	Bedtime				
Notes :					
Date	**Meal**	**Time**	**Before**	**After**	**Med/Insulin**
THU	Breakfast				
	Lunch				
	Dinner				
	Bedtime				
Notes :					

Date	Meal	Time	Before	After	Med/Insulin
FRI	Breakfast				
	Lunch				
	Dinner				
	Bedtime				

Notes :

Date	Meal	Time	Before	After	Med/Insulin
SAT	Breakfast				
	Lunch				
	Dinner				
	Bedtime				

Notes :

Date	Meal	Time	Before	After	Med/Insulin
SUN	Breakfast				
	Lunch				
	Dinner				
	Bedtime				

Notes :

Notes :

Week :				Weight :		
Date	Meal	Time	Before	After	Med/Insulin
MON	Breakfast				
	Lunch				
	Dinner				
	Bedtime				

Notes :

Date	Meal	Time	Before	After	Med/Insulin
TUE	Breakfast				
	Lunch				
	Dinner				
	Bedtime				

Notes :

Date	Meal	Time	Before	After	Med/Insulin
WED	Breakfast				
	Lunch				
	Dinner				
	Bedtime				

Notes :

Date	Meal	Time	Before	After	Med/Insulin
THU	Breakfast				
	Lunch				
	Dinner				
	Bedtime				

Notes :

Date	Meal	Time	Before	After	Med/Insulin
FRI	Breakfast				
	Lunch				
	Dinner				
	Bedtime				

Notes :

Date	Meal	Time	Before	After	Med/Insulin
SAT	Breakfast				
	Lunch				
	Dinner				
	Bedtime				

Notes :

Date	Meal	Time	Before	After	Med/Insulin
SUN	Breakfast				
	Lunch				
	Dinner				
	Bedtime				

Notes :

Notes :

- -

Week :				Weight :	
Date	Meal	Time	Before	After	Med/Insulin
MON	Breakfast				
	Lunch				
	Dinner				
	Bedtime				
Notes :					

Date	Meal	Time	Before	After	Med/Insulin
TUE	Breakfast				
	Lunch				
	Dinner				
	Bedtime				
Notes :					

Date	Meal	Time	Before	After	Med/Insulin
WED	Breakfast				
	Lunch				
	Dinner				
	Bedtime				
Notes :					

Date	Meal	Time	Before	After	Med/Insulin
THU	Breakfast				
	Lunch				
	Dinner				
	Bedtime				
Notes :					

Date	Meal	Time	Before	After	Med/Insulin
FRI	Breakfast				
	Lunch				
	Dinner				
	Bedtime				

Notes :

Date	Meal	Time	Before	After	Med/Insulin
SAT	Breakfast				
	Lunch				
	Dinner				
	Bedtime				

Notes :

Date	Meal	Time	Before	After	Med/Insulin
SUN	Breakfast				
	Lunch				
	Dinner				
	Bedtime				

Notes :

Notes :

- -

- -

- -

- -

- -

- -

- -

Week :				Weight :	

Date	Meal	Time	Before	After	Med/Insulin
MON	Breakfast				
	Lunch				
	Dinner				
	Bedtime				

Notes :

Date	Meal	Time	Before	After	Med/Insulin
TUE	Breakfast				
	Lunch				
	Dinner				
	Bedtime				

Notes :

Date	Meal	Time	Before	After	Med/Insulin
WED	Breakfast				
	Lunch				
	Dinner				
	Bedtime				

Notes :

Date	Meal	Time	Before	After	Med/Insulin
THU	Breakfast				
	Lunch				
	Dinner				
	Bedtime				

Notes :

Date	Meal	Time	Before	After	Med/Insulin
FRI	Breakfast				
	Lunch				
	Dinner				
	Bedtime				

Notes :

Date	Meal	Time	Before	After	Med/Insulin
SAT	Breakfast				
	Lunch				
	Dinner				
	Bedtime				

Notes :

Date	Meal	Time	Before	After	Med/Insulin
SUN	Breakfast				
	Lunch				
	Dinner				
	Bedtime				

Notes :

Notes :

- -
- -
- -
- -
- -
- -
- -
- -

Week :				Weight :		
Date	Meal	Time	Before	After	Med/Insulin	
MON	Breakfast					
	Lunch					
	Dinner					
	Bedtime					

Notes :

Date	Meal	Time	Before	After	Med/Insulin	
TUE	Breakfast					
	Lunch					
	Dinner					
	Bedtime					

Notes :

Date	Meal	Time	Before	After	Med/Insulin	
WED	Breakfast					
	Lunch					
	Dinner					
	Bedtime					

Notes :

Date	Meal	Time	Before	After	Med/Insulin	
THU	Breakfast					
	Lunch					
	Dinner					
	Bedtime					

Notes :

Date	Meal	Time	Before	After	Med/Insulin
FRI	Breakfast				
	Lunch				
	Dinner				
	Bedtime				

Notes :

Date	Meal	Time	Before	After	Med/Insulin
SAT	Breakfast				
	Lunch				
	Dinner				
	Bedtime				

Notes :

Date	Meal	Time	Before	After	Med/Insulin
SUN	Breakfast				
	Lunch				
	Dinner				
	Bedtime				

Notes :

Notes :

Week :				Weight :	

Date	Meal	Time	Before	After	Med/Insulin
MON	Breakfast				
	Lunch				
	Dinner				
	Bedtime				

Notes :

Date	Meal	Time	Before	After	Med/Insulin
TUE	Breakfast				
	Lunch				
	Dinner				
	Bedtime				

Notes :

Date	Meal	Time	Before	After	Med/Insulin
WED	Breakfast				
	Lunch				
	Dinner				
	Bedtime				

Notes :

Date	Meal	Time	Before	After	Med/Insulin
THU	Breakfast				
	Lunch				
	Dinner				
	Bedtime				

Notes :

Date	Meal	Time	Before	After	Med/Insulin
FRI	Breakfast				
	Lunch				
	Dinner				
	Bedtime				

Notes :

Date	Meal	Time	Before	After	Med/Insulin
SAT	Breakfast				
	Lunch				
	Dinner				
	Bedtime				

Notes :

Date	Meal	Time	Before	After	Med/Insulin
SUN	Breakfast				
	Lunch				
	Dinner				
	Bedtime				

Notes :

Notes :

Week :				Weight :	

Date	Meal	Time	Before	After	Med/Insulin
MON	Breakfast				
	Lunch				
	Dinner				
	Bedtime				

Notes :

Date	Meal	Time	Before	After	Med/Insulin
TUE	Breakfast				
	Lunch				
	Dinner				
	Bedtime				

Notes :

Date	Meal	Time	Before	After	Med/Insulin
WED	Breakfast				
	Lunch				
	Dinner				
	Bedtime				

Notes :

Date	Meal	Time	Before	After	Med/Insulin
THU	Breakfast				
	Lunch				
	Dinner				
	Bedtime				

Notes :

Date	Meal	Time	Before	After	Med/Insulin
FRI	Breakfast				
	Lunch				
	Dinner				
	Bedtime				
Notes :					

Date	Meal	Time	Before	After	Med/Insulin
SAT	Breakfast				
	Lunch				
	Dinner				
	Bedtime				
Notes :					

Date	Meal	Time	Before	After	Med/Insulin
SUN	Breakfast				
	Lunch				
	Dinner				
	Bedtime				
Notes :					

Notes :

Week :				Weight :	
Date	Meal	Time	Before	After	Med/Insulin
MON	Breakfast				
	Lunch				
	Dinner				
	Bedtime				

Notes :

Date	Meal	Time	Before	After	Med/Insulin
TUE	Breakfast				
	Lunch				
	Dinner				
	Bedtime				

Notes :

Date	Meal	Time	Before	After	Med/Insulin
WED	Breakfast				
	Lunch				
	Dinner				
	Bedtime				

Notes :

Date	Meal	Time	Before	After	Med/Insulin
THU	Breakfast				
	Lunch				
	Dinner				
	Bedtime				

Notes :

Date	Meal	Time	Before	After	Med/Insulin
FRI	Breakfast				
	Lunch				
	Dinner				
	Bedtime				
Notes :					

Date	Meal	Time	Before	After	Med/Insulin
SAT	Breakfast				
	Lunch				
	Dinner				
	Bedtime				
Notes :					

Date	Meal	Time	Before	After	Med/Insulin
SUN	Breakfast				
	Lunch				
	Dinner				
	Bedtime				
Notes :					

Notes :

Week :				Weight :	

Date	Meal	Time	Before	After	Med/Insulin
MON	Breakfast				
	Lunch				
	Dinner				
	Bedtime				

Notes :

Date	Meal	Time	Before	After	Med/Insulin
TUE	Breakfast				
	Lunch				
	Dinner				
	Bedtime				

Notes :

Date	Meal	Time	Before	After	Med/Insulin
WED	Breakfast				
	Lunch				
	Dinner				
	Bedtime				

Notes :

Date	Meal	Time	Before	After	Med/Insulin
THU	Breakfast				
	Lunch				
	Dinner				
	Bedtime				

Notes :

Date	Meal	Time	Before	After	Med/Insulin
FRI	Breakfast				
	Lunch				
	Dinner				
	Bedtime				

Notes :

Date	Meal	Time	Before	After	Med/Insulin
SAT	Breakfast				
	Lunch				
	Dinner				
	Bedtime				

Notes :

Date	Meal	Time	Before	After	Med/Insulin
SUN	Breakfast				
	Lunch				
	Dinner				
	Bedtime				

Notes :

Notes :

Week :				Weight :		

Date	Meal	Time	Before	After	Med/Insulin
MON	Breakfast				
	Lunch				
	Dinner				
	Bedtime				

Notes :

Date	Meal	Time	Before	After	Med/Insulin
TUE	Breakfast				
	Lunch				
	Dinner				
	Bedtime				

Notes :

Date	Meal	Time	Before	After	Med/Insulin
WED	Breakfast				
	Lunch				
	Dinner				
	Bedtime				

Notes :

Date	Meal	Time	Before	After	Med/Insulin
THU	Breakfast				
	Lunch				
	Dinner				
	Bedtime				

Notes :

Date	Meal	Time	Before	After	Med/Insulin
FRI	Breakfast				
	Lunch				
	Dinner				
	Bedtime				

Notes :

Date	Meal	Time	Before	After	Med/Insulin
SAT	Breakfast				
	Lunch				
	Dinner				
	Bedtime				

Notes :

Date	Meal	Time	Before	After	Med/Insulin
SUN	Breakfast				
	Lunch				
	Dinner				
	Bedtime				

Notes :

Notes :

Week :				Weight :	
Date	Meal	Time	Before	After	Med/Insulin
MON	Breakfast				
	Lunch				
	Dinner				
	Bedtime				

Notes :

Date	Meal	Time	Before	After	Med/Insulin
TUE	Breakfast				
	Lunch				
	Dinner				
	Bedtime				

Notes :

Date	Meal	Time	Before	After	Med/Insulin
WED	Breakfast				
	Lunch				
	Dinner				
	Bedtime				

Notes :

Date	Meal	Time	Before	After	Med/Insulin
THU	Breakfast				
	Lunch				
	Dinner				
	Bedtime				

Notes :

Date	Meal	Time	Before	After	Med/Insulin
FRI	Breakfast				
	Lunch				
	Dinner				
	Bedtime				

Notes :

Date	Meal	Time	Before	After	Med/Insulin
SAT	Breakfast				
	Lunch				
	Dinner				
	Bedtime				

Notes :

Date	Meal	Time	Before	After	Med/Insulin
SUN	Breakfast				
	Lunch				
	Dinner				
	Bedtime				

Notes :

Notes :
- -
- -
- -
- -
- -
- -
- -

Week :				Weight :	

Date	Meal	Time	Before	After	Med/Insulin
MON	Breakfast				
	Lunch				
	Dinner				
	Bedtime				

Notes :

Date	Meal	Time	Before	After	Med/Insulin
TUE	Breakfast				
	Lunch				
	Dinner				
	Bedtime				

Notes :

Date	Meal	Time	Before	After	Med/Insulin
WED	Breakfast				
	Lunch				
	Dinner				
	Bedtime				

Notes :

Date	Meal	Time	Before	After	Med/Insulin
THU	Breakfast				
	Lunch				
	Dinner				
	Bedtime				

Notes :

Date	Meal	Time	Before	After	Med/Insulin
FRI	Breakfast				
	Lunch				
	Dinner				
	Bedtime				

Notes :

Date	Meal	Time	Before	After	Med/Insulin
SAT	Breakfast				
	Lunch				
	Dinner				
	Bedtime				

Notes :

Date	Meal	Time	Before	After	Med/Insulin
SUN	Breakfast				
	Lunch				
	Dinner				
	Bedtime				

Notes :

Notes :

- -
- -
- -
- -
- -
- -
- -
- -

Week :				Weight :	
Date	**Meal**	**Time**	**Before**	**After**	**Med/Insulin**
MON	Breakfast				
	Lunch				
	Dinner				
	Bedtime				

Notes :

Date	**Meal**	**Time**	**Before**	**After**	**Med/Insulin**
TUE	Breakfast				
	Lunch				
	Dinner				
	Bedtime				

Notes :

Date	**Meal**	**Time**	**Before**	**After**	**Med/Insulin**
WED	Breakfast				
	Lunch				
	Dinner				
	Bedtime				

Notes :

Date	**Meal**	**Time**	**Before**	**After**	**Med/Insulin**
THU	Breakfast				
	Lunch				
	Dinner				
	Bedtime				

Notes :

Date	Meal	Time	Before	After	Med/Insulin
FRI	Breakfast				
	Lunch				
	Dinner				
	Bedtime				

Notes :

Date	Meal	Time	Before	After	Med/Insulin
SAT	Breakfast				
	Lunch				
	Dinner				
	Bedtime				

Notes :

Date	Meal	Time	Before	After	Med/Insulin
SUN	Breakfast				
	Lunch				
	Dinner				
	Bedtime				

Notes :

Notes :

- -

- -

- -

- -

- -

- -

Week :				Weight :	
Date	Meal	Time	Before	After	Med/Insulin
MON	Breakfast				
	Lunch				
	Dinner				
	Bedtime				
Notes :					

Date	Meal	Time	Before	After	Med/Insulin
TUE	Breakfast				
	Lunch				
	Dinner				
	Bedtime				
Notes :					

Date	Meal	Time	Before	After	Med/Insulin
WED	Breakfast				
	Lunch				
	Dinner				
	Bedtime				
Notes :					

Date	Meal	Time	Before	After	Med/Insulin
THU	Breakfast				
	Lunch				
	Dinner				
	Bedtime				
Notes :					

Date	Meal	Time	Before	After	Med/Insulin
FRI	Breakfast				
	Lunch				
	Dinner				
	Bedtime				

Notes :

Date	Meal	Time	Before	After	Med/Insulin
SAT	Breakfast				
	Lunch				
	Dinner				
	Bedtime				

Notes :

Date	Meal	Time	Before	After	Med/Insulin
SUN	Breakfast				
	Lunch				
	Dinner				
	Bedtime				

Notes :

Notes :

- -
- -
- -
- -
- -
- -
- -
- -

Week :				Weight :	
Date	**Meal**	**Time**	**Before**	**After**	**Med/Insulin**
MON	Breakfast				
	Lunch				
	Dinner				
	Bedtime				

Notes :

Date	**Meal**	**Time**	**Before**	**After**	**Med/Insulin**
TUE	Breakfast				
	Lunch				
	Dinner				
	Bedtime				

Notes :

Date	**Meal**	**Time**	**Before**	**After**	**Med/Insulin**
WED	Breakfast				
	Lunch				
	Dinner				
	Bedtime				

Notes :

Date	**Meal**	**Time**	**Before**	**After**	**Med/Insulin**
THU	Breakfast				
	Lunch				
	Dinner				
	Bedtime				

Notes :

Date	Meal	Time	Before	After	Med/Insulin
FRI	Breakfast				
	Lunch				
	Dinner				
	Bedtime				

Notes :

Date	Meal	Time	Before	After	Med/Insulin
SAT	Breakfast				
	Lunch				
	Dinner				
	Bedtime				

Notes :

Date	Meal	Time	Before	After	Med/Insulin
SUN	Breakfast				
	Lunch				
	Dinner				
	Bedtime				

Notes :

Notes :

Week :				Weight :		
Date	Meal	Time	Before	After	Med/Insulin	
MON	Breakfast					
	Lunch					
	Dinner					
	Bedtime					
Notes :						

Date	Meal	Time	Before	After	Med/Insulin	
TUE	Breakfast					
	Lunch					
	Dinner					
	Bedtime					
Notes :						

Date	Meal	Time	Before	After	Med/Insulin	
WED	Breakfast					
	Lunch					
	Dinner					
	Bedtime					
Notes :						

Date	Meal	Time	Before	After	Med/Insulin	
THU	Breakfast					
	Lunch					
	Dinner					
	Bedtime					
Notes :						

Date	Meal	Time	Before	After	Med/Insulin
FRI	Breakfast				
	Lunch				
	Dinner				
	Bedtime				

Notes :

Date	Meal	Time	Before	After	Med/Insulin
SAT	Breakfast				
	Lunch				
	Dinner				
	Bedtime				

Notes :

Date	Meal	Time	Before	After	Med/Insulin
SUN	Breakfast				
	Lunch				
	Dinner				
	Bedtime				

Notes :

Notes :

Week :				Weight :	

Date	Meal	Time	Before	After	Med/Insulin
MON	Breakfast				
	Lunch				
	Dinner				
	Bedtime				

Notes :

Date	Meal	Time	Before	After	Med/Insulin
TUE	Breakfast				
	Lunch				
	Dinner				
	Bedtime				

Notes :

Date	Meal	Time	Before	After	Med/Insulin
WED	Breakfast				
	Lunch				
	Dinner				
	Bedtime				

Notes :

Date	Meal	Time	Before	After	Med/Insulin
THU	Breakfast				
	Lunch				
	Dinner				
	Bedtime				

Notes :

Date	Meal	Time	Before	After	Med/Insulin
FRI	Breakfast				
	Lunch				
	Dinner				
	Bedtime				

Notes :

Date	Meal	Time	Before	After	Med/Insulin
SAT	Breakfast				
	Lunch				
	Dinner				
	Bedtime				

Notes :

Date	Meal	Time	Before	After	Med/Insulin
SUN	Breakfast				
	Lunch				
	Dinner				
	Bedtime				

Notes :

Notes :

Week :				Weight :	
Date	Meal	Time	Before	After	Med/Insulin
MON	Breakfast				
	Lunch				
	Dinner				
	Bedtime				
Notes :					

Date	Meal	Time	Before	After	Med/Insulin
TUE	Breakfast				
	Lunch				
	Dinner				
	Bedtime				
Notes :					

Date	Meal	Time	Before	After	Med/Insulin
WED	Breakfast				
	Lunch				
	Dinner				
	Bedtime				
Notes :					

Date	Meal	Time	Before	After	Med/Insulin
THU	Breakfast				
	Lunch				
	Dinner				
	Bedtime				
Notes :					

Date	Meal	Time	Before	After	Med/Insulin
FRI	Breakfast				
	Lunch				
	Dinner				
	Bedtime				

Notes :

Date	Meal	Time	Before	After	Med/Insulin
SAT	Breakfast				
	Lunch				
	Dinner				
	Bedtime				

Notes :

Date	Meal	Time	Before	After	Med/Insulin
SUN	Breakfast				
	Lunch				
	Dinner				
	Bedtime				

Notes :

Notes :

Week :				Weight :	
Date	Meal	Time	Before	After	Med/Insulin
MON	Breakfast				
	Lunch				
	Dinner				
	Bedtime				
Notes :					

Date	Meal	Time	Before	After	Med/Insulin
TUE	Breakfast				
	Lunch				
	Dinner				
	Bedtime				
Notes :					

Date	Meal	Time	Before	After	Med/Insulin
WED	Breakfast				
	Lunch				
	Dinner				
	Bedtime				
Notes :					

Date	Meal	Time	Before	After	Med/Insulin
THU	Breakfast				
	Lunch				
	Dinner				
	Bedtime				
Notes :					

Date	Meal	Time	Before	After	Med/Insulin
FRI	Breakfast				
	Lunch				
	Dinner				
	Bedtime				

Notes :

Date	Meal	Time	Before	After	Med/Insulin
SAT	Breakfast				
	Lunch				
	Dinner				
	Bedtime				

Notes :

Date	Meal	Time	Before	After	Med/Insulin
SUN	Breakfast				
	Lunch				
	Dinner				
	Bedtime				

Notes :

Notes :

Week :				Weight :	
Date	Meal	Time	Before	After	Med/Insulin
MON	Breakfast				
	Lunch				
	Dinner				
	Bedtime				

Notes :

Date	Meal	Time	Before	After	Med/Insulin
TUE	Breakfast				
	Lunch				
	Dinner				
	Bedtime				

Notes :

Date	Meal	Time	Before	After	Med/Insulin
WED	Breakfast				
	Lunch				
	Dinner				
	Bedtime				

Notes :

Date	Meal	Time	Before	After	Med/Insulin
THU	Breakfast				
	Lunch				
	Dinner				
	Bedtime				

Notes :

Date	Meal	Time	Before	After	Med/Insulin
FRI	Breakfast				
	Lunch				
	Dinner				
	Bedtime				

Notes :

Date	Meal	Time	Before	After	Med/Insulin
SAT	Breakfast				
	Lunch				
	Dinner				
	Bedtime				

Notes :

Date	Meal	Time	Before	After	Med/Insulin
SUN	Breakfast				
	Lunch				
	Dinner				
	Bedtime				

Notes :

Notes :

Week :				Weight :	
Date	Meal	Time	Before	After	Med/Insulin
MON	Breakfast				
	Lunch				
	Dinner				
	Bedtime				

Notes :

Date	Meal	Time	Before	After	Med/Insulin
TUE	Breakfast				
	Lunch				
	Dinner				
	Bedtime				

Notes :

Date	Meal	Time	Before	After	Med/Insulin
WED	Breakfast				
	Lunch				
	Dinner				
	Bedtime				

Notes :

Date	Meal	Time	Before	After	Med/Insulin
THU	Breakfast				
	Lunch				
	Dinner				
	Bedtime				

Notes :

Date	Meal	Time	Before	After	Med/Insulin
FRI	Breakfast				
	Lunch				
	Dinner				
	Bedtime				

Notes :

Date	Meal	Time	Before	After	Med/Insulin
SAT	Breakfast				
	Lunch				
	Dinner				
	Bedtime				

Notes :

Date	Meal	Time	Before	After	Med/Insulin
SUN	Breakfast				
	Lunch				
	Dinner				
	Bedtime				

Notes :

Notes :

Week :				Weight :	
Date	Meal	Time	Before	After	Med/Insulin
MON	Breakfast				
	Lunch				
	Dinner				
	Bedtime				
Notes :					

Date	Meal	Time	Before	After	Med/Insulin
TUE	Breakfast				
	Lunch				
	Dinner				
	Bedtime				
Notes :					

Date	Meal	Time	Before	After	Med/Insulin
WED	Breakfast				
	Lunch				
	Dinner				
	Bedtime				
Notes :					

Date	Meal	Time	Before	After	Med/Insulin
THU	Breakfast				
	Lunch				
	Dinner				
	Bedtime				
Notes :					

Date	Meal	Time	Before	After	Med/Insulin
FRI	Breakfast				
	Lunch				
	Dinner				
	Bedtime				

Notes :

Date	Meal	Time	Before	After	Med/Insulin
SAT	Breakfast				
	Lunch				
	Dinner				
	Bedtime				

Notes :

Date	Meal	Time	Before	After	Med/Insulin
SUN	Breakfast				
	Lunch				
	Dinner				
	Bedtime				

Notes :

Notes :

Week :				Weight :	
Date	Meal	Time	Before	After	Med/Insulin
MON	Breakfast				
	Lunch				
	Dinner				
	Bedtime				

Notes :

Date	Meal	Time	Before	After	Med/Insulin
TUE	Breakfast				
	Lunch				
	Dinner				
	Bedtime				

Notes :

Date	Meal	Time	Before	After	Med/Insulin
WED	Breakfast				
	Lunch				
	Dinner				
	Bedtime				

Notes :

Date	Meal	Time	Before	After	Med/Insulin
THU	Breakfast				
	Lunch				
	Dinner				
	Bedtime				

Notes :

Date	Meal	Time	Before	After	Med/Insulin
FRI	Breakfast				
	Lunch				
	Dinner				
	Bedtime				

Notes :

Date	Meal	Time	Before	After	Med/Insulin
SAT	Breakfast				
	Lunch				
	Dinner				
	Bedtime				

Notes :

Date	Meal	Time	Before	After	Med/Insulin
SUN	Breakfast				
	Lunch				
	Dinner				
	Bedtime				

Notes :

Notes :

Week :				Weight :	

Date	Meal	Time	Before	After	Med/Insulin
MON	Breakfast				
	Lunch				
	Dinner				
	Bedtime				

Notes :

Date	Meal	Time	Before	After	Med/Insulin
TUE	Breakfast				
	Lunch				
	Dinner				
	Bedtime				

Notes :

Date	Meal	Time	Before	After	Med/Insulin
WED	Breakfast				
	Lunch				
	Dinner				
	Bedtime				

Notes :

Date	Meal	Time	Before	After	Med/Insulin
THU	Breakfast				
	Lunch				
	Dinner				
	Bedtime				

Notes :

Date	Meal	Time	Before	After	Med/Insulin
FRI	Breakfast				
	Lunch				
	Dinner				
	Bedtime				
Notes :					

Date	Meal	Time	Before	After	Med/Insulin
SAT	Breakfast				
	Lunch				
	Dinner				
	Bedtime				
Notes :					

Date	Meal	Time	Before	After	Med/Insulin
SUN	Breakfast				
	Lunch				
	Dinner				
	Bedtime				
Notes :					

Notes :

Week :				Weight :	
Date	Meal	Time	Before	After	Med/Insulin
MON	Breakfast				
	Lunch				
	Dinner				
	Bedtime				

Notes :

Date	Meal	Time	Before	After	Med/Insulin
TUE	Breakfast				
	Lunch				
	Dinner				
	Bedtime				

Notes :

Date	Meal	Time	Before	After	Med/Insulin
WED	Breakfast				
	Lunch				
	Dinner				
	Bedtime				

Notes :

Date	Meal	Time	Before	After	Med/Insulin
THU	Breakfast				
	Lunch				
	Dinner				
	Bedtime				

Notes :

Date	Meal	Time	Before	After	Med/Insulin
FRI	Breakfast				
	Lunch				
	Dinner				
	Bedtime				

Notes :

Date	Meal	Time	Before	After	Med/Insulin
SAT	Breakfast				
	Lunch				
	Dinner				
	Bedtime				

Notes :

Date	Meal	Time	Before	After	Med/Insulin
SUN	Breakfast				
	Lunch				
	Dinner				
	Bedtime				

Notes :

Notes :

Week :				Weight :	
Date	**Meal**	**Time**	**Before**	**After**	**Med/Insulin**
MON	Breakfast				
	Lunch				
	Dinner				
	Bedtime				
Notes :					
Date	**Meal**	**Time**	**Before**	**After**	**Med/Insulin**
TUE	Breakfast				
	Lunch				
	Dinner				
	Bedtime				
Notes :					
Date	**Meal**	**Time**	**Before**	**After**	**Med/Insulin**
WED	Breakfast				
	Lunch				
	Dinner				
	Bedtime				
Notes :					
Date	**Meal**	**Time**	**Before**	**After**	**Med/Insulin**
THU	Breakfast				
	Lunch				
	Dinner				
	Bedtime				
Notes :					

Date	Meal	Time	Before	After	Med/Insulin
FRI	Breakfast				
	Lunch				
	Dinner				
	Bedtime				

Notes :

Date	Meal	Time	Before	After	Med/Insulin
SAT	Breakfast				
	Lunch				
	Dinner				
	Bedtime				

Notes :

Date	Meal	Time	Before	After	Med/Insulin
SUN	Breakfast				
	Lunch				
	Dinner				
	Bedtime				

Notes :

Notes :

- -
- -
- -
- -
- -
- -
- -

Week :				Weight :	
Date	Meal	Time	Before	After	Med/Insulin
MON	Breakfast				
	Lunch				
	Dinner				
	Bedtime				

Notes :

Date	Meal	Time	Before	After	Med/Insulin
TUE	Breakfast				
	Lunch				
	Dinner				
	Bedtime				

Notes :

Date	Meal	Time	Before	After	Med/Insulin
WED	Breakfast				
	Lunch				
	Dinner				
	Bedtime				

Notes :

Date	Meal	Time	Before	After	Med/Insulin
THU	Breakfast				
	Lunch				
	Dinner				
	Bedtime				

Notes :

Date	Meal	Time	Before	After	Med/Insulin
FRI	Breakfast				
	Lunch				
	Dinner				
	Bedtime				

Notes :

Date	Meal	Time	Before	After	Med/Insulin
SAT	Breakfast				
	Lunch				
	Dinner				
	Bedtime				

Notes :

Date	Meal	Time	Before	After	Med/Insulin
SUN	Breakfast				
	Lunch				
	Dinner				
	Bedtime				

Notes :

Notes :

Week :				Weight :	
Date	Meal	Time	Before	After	Med/Insulin
MON	Breakfast				
	Lunch				
	Dinner				
	Bedtime				
Notes :					

Date	Meal	Time	Before	After	Med/Insulin
TUE	Breakfast				
	Lunch				
	Dinner				
	Bedtime				
Notes :					

Date	Meal	Time	Before	After	Med/Insulin
WED	Breakfast				
	Lunch				
	Dinner				
	Bedtime				
Notes :					

Date	Meal	Time	Before	After	Med/Insulin
THU	Breakfast				
	Lunch				
	Dinner				
	Bedtime				
Notes :					

Date	Meal	Time	Before	After	Med/Insulin
FRI	Breakfast				
	Lunch				
	Dinner				
	Bedtime				
Notes :					

Date	Meal	Time	Before	After	Med/Insulin
SAT	Breakfast				
	Lunch				
	Dinner				
	Bedtime				
Notes :					

Date	Meal	Time	Before	After	Med/Insulin
SUN	Breakfast				
	Lunch				
	Dinner				
	Bedtime				
Notes :					

Notes :

Week :				Weight :	

Date	Meal	Time	Before	After	Med/Insulin
MON	Breakfast				
	Lunch				
	Dinner				
	Bedtime				

Notes :

Date	Meal	Time	Before	After	Med/Insulin
TUE	Breakfast				
	Lunch				
	Dinner				
	Bedtime				

Notes :

Date	Meal	Time	Before	After	Med/Insulin
WED	Breakfast				
	Lunch				
	Dinner				
	Bedtime				

Notes :

Date	Meal	Time	Before	After	Med/Insulin
THU	Breakfast				
	Lunch				
	Dinner				
	Bedtime				

Notes :

Date	Meal	Time	Before	After	Med/Insulin
FRI	Breakfast				
	Lunch				
	Dinner				
	Bedtime				

Notes :

Date	Meal	Time	Before	After	Med/Insulin
SAT	Breakfast				
	Lunch				
	Dinner				
	Bedtime				

Notes :

Date	Meal	Time	Before	After	Med/Insulin
SUN	Breakfast				
	Lunch				
	Dinner				
	Bedtime				

Notes :

Notes :

Week :				Weight :	
Date	Meal	Time	Before	After	Med/Insulin
MON	Breakfast				
	Lunch				
	Dinner				
	Bedtime				

Notes :

Date	Meal	Time	Before	After	Med/Insulin
TUE	Breakfast				
	Lunch				
	Dinner				
	Bedtime				

Notes :

Date	Meal	Time	Before	After	Med/Insulin
WED	Breakfast				
	Lunch				
	Dinner				
	Bedtime				

Notes :

Date	Meal	Time	Before	After	Med/Insulin
THU	Breakfast				
	Lunch				
	Dinner				
	Bedtime				

Notes :

Date	Meal	Time	Before	After	Med/Insulin
FRI	Breakfast				
	Lunch				
	Dinner				
	Bedtime				

Notes :

Date	Meal	Time	Before	After	Med/Insulin
SAT	Breakfast				
	Lunch				
	Dinner				
	Bedtime				

Notes :

Date	Meal	Time	Before	After	Med/Insulin
SUN	Breakfast				
	Lunch				
	Dinner				
	Bedtime				

Notes :

Notes :

Week :				Weight :	
Date	Meal	Time	Before	After	Med/Insulin
MON	Breakfast				
	Lunch				
	Dinner				
	Bedtime				

Notes :

Date	Meal	Time	Before	After	Med/Insulin
TUE	Breakfast				
	Lunch				
	Dinner				
	Bedtime				

Notes :

Date	Meal	Time	Before	After	Med/Insulin
WED	Breakfast				
	Lunch				
	Dinner				
	Bedtime				

Notes :

Date	Meal	Time	Before	After	Med/Insulin
THU	Breakfast				
	Lunch				
	Dinner				
	Bedtime				

Notes :

Date	Meal	Time	Before	After	Med/Insulin
FRI	Breakfast				
	Lunch				
	Dinner				
	Bedtime				

Notes :

Date	Meal	Time	Before	After	Med/Insulin
SAT	Breakfast				
	Lunch				
	Dinner				
	Bedtime				

Notes :

Date	Meal	Time	Before	After	Med/Insulin
SUN	Breakfast				
	Lunch				
	Dinner				
	Bedtime				

Notes :

Notes :

Week :				Weight :	
Date	**Meal**	**Time**	**Before**	**After**	**Med/Insulin**
MON	Breakfast				
	Lunch				
	Dinner				
	Bedtime				
Notes :					

Date	**Meal**	**Time**	**Before**	**After**	**Med/Insulin**
TUE	Breakfast				
	Lunch				
	Dinner				
	Bedtime				
Notes :					

Date	**Meal**	**Time**	**Before**	**After**	**Med/Insulin**
WED	Breakfast				
	Lunch				
	Dinner				
	Bedtime				
Notes :					

Date	**Meal**	**Time**	**Before**	**After**	**Med/Insulin**
THU	Breakfast				
	Lunch				
	Dinner				
	Bedtime				
Notes :					

Date	Meal	Time	Before	After	Med/Insulin
FRI	Breakfast				
	Lunch				
	Dinner				
	Bedtime				

Notes :

Date	Meal	Time	Before	After	Med/Insulin
SAT	Breakfast				
	Lunch				
	Dinner				
	Bedtime				

Notes :

Date	Meal	Time	Before	After	Med/Insulin
SUN	Breakfast				
	Lunch				
	Dinner				
	Bedtime				

Notes :

Notes :

- -
- -
- -
- -
- -
- -
- -
- -

Week :				Weight :	

Date	Meal	Time	Before	After	Med/Insulin
MON	Breakfast				
	Lunch				
	Dinner				
	Bedtime				

Notes :

Date	Meal	Time	Before	After	Med/Insulin
TUE	Breakfast				
	Lunch				
	Dinner				
	Bedtime				

Notes :

Date	Meal	Time	Before	After	Med/Insulin
WED	Breakfast				
	Lunch				
	Dinner				
	Bedtime				

Notes :

Date	Meal	Time	Before	After	Med/Insulin
THU	Breakfast				
	Lunch				
	Dinner				
	Bedtime				

Notes :

Date	Meal	Time	Before	After	Med/Insulin
FRI	Breakfast				
	Lunch				
	Dinner				
	Bedtime				

Notes :

Date	Meal	Time	Before	After	Med/Insulin
SAT	Breakfast				
	Lunch				
	Dinner				
	Bedtime				

Notes :

Date	Meal	Time	Before	After	Med/Insulin
SUN	Breakfast				
	Lunch				
	Dinner				
	Bedtime				

Notes :

Notes :

Week :				Weight :	

Date	Meal	Time	Before	After	Med/Insulin
MON	Breakfast				
	Lunch				
	Dinner				
	Bedtime				

Notes :

Date	Meal	Time	Before	After	Med/Insulin
TUE	Breakfast				
	Lunch				
	Dinner				
	Bedtime				

Notes :

Date	Meal	Time	Before	After	Med/Insulin
WED	Breakfast				
	Lunch				
	Dinner				
	Bedtime				

Notes :

Date	Meal	Time	Before	After	Med/Insulin
THU	Breakfast				
	Lunch				
	Dinner				
	Bedtime				

Notes :

Date	Meal	Time	Before	After	Med/Insulin
FRI	Breakfast				
	Lunch				
	Dinner				
	Bedtime				

Notes :

Date	Meal	Time	Before	After	Med/Insulin
SAT	Breakfast				
	Lunch				
	Dinner				
	Bedtime				

Notes :

Date	Meal	Time	Before	After	Med/Insulin
SUN	Breakfast				
	Lunch				
	Dinner				
	Bedtime				

Notes :

Notes :

- -
- -
- -
- -
- -
- -
- -
- -

Week :				Weight :		
Date	Meal	Time	Before	After	Med/Insulin
MON	Breakfast				
	Lunch				
	Dinner				
	Bedtime				
Notes :					

Date	Meal	Time	Before	After	Med/Insulin
TUE	Breakfast				
	Lunch				
	Dinner				
	Bedtime				
Notes :					

Date	Meal	Time	Before	After	Med/Insulin
WED	Breakfast				
	Lunch				
	Dinner				
	Bedtime				
Notes :					

Date	Meal	Time	Before	After	Med/Insulin
THU	Breakfast				
	Lunch				
	Dinner				
	Bedtime				
Notes :					

Date	Meal	Time	Before	After	Med/Insulin
FRI	Breakfast				
	Lunch				
	Dinner				
	Bedtime				

Notes :

Date	Meal	Time	Before	After	Med/Insulin
SAT	Breakfast				
	Lunch				
	Dinner				
	Bedtime				

Notes :

Date	Meal	Time	Before	After	Med/Insulin
SUN	Breakfast				
	Lunch				
	Dinner				
	Bedtime				

Notes :

Notes :

Week :				Weight :	
Date	Meal	Time	Before	After	Med/Insulin
MON	Breakfast				
	Lunch				
	Dinner				
	Bedtime				
Notes :					

Date	Meal	Time	Before	After	Med/Insulin
TUE	Breakfast				
	Lunch				
	Dinner				
	Bedtime				
Notes :					

Date	Meal	Time	Before	After	Med/Insulin
WED	Breakfast				
	Lunch				
	Dinner				
	Bedtime				
Notes :					

Date	Meal	Time	Before	After	Med/Insulin
THU	Breakfast				
	Lunch				
	Dinner				
	Bedtime				
Notes :					

Date	Meal	Time	Before	After	Med/Insulin
FRI	Breakfast				
	Lunch				
	Dinner				
	Bedtime				

Notes :

Date	Meal	Time	Before	After	Med/Insulin
SAT	Breakfast				
	Lunch				
	Dinner				
	Bedtime				

Notes :

Date	Meal	Time	Before	After	Med/Insulin
SUN	Breakfast				
	Lunch				
	Dinner				
	Bedtime				

Notes :

Notes :

Week :				Weight :	

Date	Meal	Time	Before	After	Med/Insulin
MON	Breakfast				
	Lunch				
	Dinner				
	Bedtime				

Notes :

Date	Meal	Time	Before	After	Med/Insulin
TUE	Breakfast				
	Lunch				
	Dinner				
	Bedtime				

Notes :

Date	Meal	Time	Before	After	Med/Insulin
WED	Breakfast				
	Lunch				
	Dinner				
	Bedtime				

Notes :

Date	Meal	Time	Before	After	Med/Insulin
THU	Breakfast				
	Lunch				
	Dinner				
	Bedtime				

Notes :

Date	Meal	Time	Before	After	Med/Insulin
FRI	Breakfast				
	Lunch				
	Dinner				
	Bedtime				

Notes :

Date	Meal	Time	Before	After	Med/Insulin
SAT	Breakfast				
	Lunch				
	Dinner				
	Bedtime				

Notes :

Date	Meal	Time	Before	After	Med/Insulin
SUN	Breakfast				
	Lunch				
	Dinner				
	Bedtime				

Notes :

Notes :

Week :				Weight :	
Date	Meal	Time	Before	After	Med/Insulin
MON	Breakfast				
	Lunch				
	Dinner				
	Bedtime				
Notes :					

Date	Meal	Time	Before	After	Med/Insulin
TUE	Breakfast				
	Lunch				
	Dinner				
	Bedtime				
Notes :					

Date	Meal	Time	Before	After	Med/Insulin
WED	Breakfast				
	Lunch				
	Dinner				
	Bedtime				
Notes :					

Date	Meal	Time	Before	After	Med/Insulin
THU	Breakfast				
	Lunch				
	Dinner				
	Bedtime				
Notes :					

Date	Meal	Time	Before	After	Med/Insulin
FRI	Breakfast				
	Lunch				
	Dinner				
	Bedtime				

Notes :

Date	Meal	Time	Before	After	Med/Insulin
SAT	Breakfast				
	Lunch				
	Dinner				
	Bedtime				

Notes :

Date	Meal	Time	Before	After	Med/Insulin
SUN	Breakfast				
	Lunch				
	Dinner				
	Bedtime				

Notes :

Notes :

- -

- -

- -

- -

- -

- -

- -

- -

Week :				Weight :	

Date	Meal	Time	Before	After	Med/Insulin
MON	Breakfast				
	Lunch				
	Dinner				
	Bedtime				

Notes :

Date	Meal	Time	Before	After	Med/Insulin
TUE	Breakfast				
	Lunch				
	Dinner				
	Bedtime				

Notes :

Date	Meal	Time	Before	After	Med/Insulin
WED	Breakfast				
	Lunch				
	Dinner				
	Bedtime				

Notes :

Date	Meal	Time	Before	After	Med/Insulin
THU	Breakfast				
	Lunch				
	Dinner				
	Bedtime				

Notes :

Date	Meal	Time	Before	After	Med/Insulin
FRI	Breakfast				
	Lunch				
	Dinner				
	Bedtime				
Notes :					

Date	Meal	Time	Before	After	Med/Insulin
SAT	Breakfast				
	Lunch				
	Dinner				
	Bedtime				
Notes :					

Date	Meal	Time	Before	After	Med/Insulin
SUN	Breakfast				
	Lunch				
	Dinner				
	Bedtime				
Notes :					

Notes :

Week :				Weight :	

Date	Meal	Time	Before	After	Med/Insulin
MON	Breakfast				
	Lunch				
	Dinner				
	Bedtime				

Notes :

Date	Meal	Time	Before	After	Med/Insulin
TUE	Breakfast				
	Lunch				
	Dinner				
	Bedtime				

Notes :

Date	Meal	Time	Before	After	Med/Insulin
WED	Breakfast				
	Lunch				
	Dinner				
	Bedtime				

Notes :

Date	Meal	Time	Before	After	Med/Insulin
THU	Breakfast				
	Lunch				
	Dinner				
	Bedtime				

Notes :

Date	Meal	Time	Before	After	Med/Insulin
FRI	Breakfast				
	Lunch				
	Dinner				
	Bedtime				
Notes :					

Date	Meal	Time	Before	After	Med/Insulin
SAT	Breakfast				
	Lunch				
	Dinner				
	Bedtime				
Notes :					

Date	Meal	Time	Before	After	Med/Insulin
SUN	Breakfast				
	Lunch				
	Dinner				
	Bedtime				
Notes :					

Notes :

Week :				Weight :	
Date	**Meal**	**Time**	**Before**	**After**	**Med/Insulin**
MON	Breakfast				
	Lunch				
	Dinner				
	Bedtime				
Notes :					

Date	**Meal**	**Time**	**Before**	**After**	**Med/Insulin**
TUE	Breakfast				
	Lunch				
	Dinner				
	Bedtime				
Notes :					

Date	**Meal**	**Time**	**Before**	**After**	**Med/Insulin**
WED	Breakfast				
	Lunch				
	Dinner				
	Bedtime				
Notes :					

Date	**Meal**	**Time**	**Before**	**After**	**Med/Insulin**
THU	Breakfast				
	Lunch				
	Dinner				
	Bedtime				
Notes :					

Date	Meal	Time	Before	After	Med/Insulin
FRI	Breakfast				
	Lunch				
	Dinner				
	Bedtime				

Notes :

Date	Meal	Time	Before	After	Med/Insulin
SAT	Breakfast				
	Lunch				
	Dinner				
	Bedtime				

Notes :

Date	Meal	Time	Before	After	Med/Insulin
SUN	Breakfast				
	Lunch				
	Dinner				
	Bedtime				

Notes :

Notes :

- -

- -

- -

- -

- -

- -

- -

- -

Week :				Weight :	
Date	Meal	Time	Before	After	Med/Insulin
MON	Breakfast				
	Lunch				
	Dinner				
	Bedtime				

Notes :

Date	Meal	Time	Before	After	Med/Insulin
TUE	Breakfast				
	Lunch				
	Dinner				
	Bedtime				

Notes :

Date	Meal	Time	Before	After	Med/Insulin
WED	Breakfast				
	Lunch				
	Dinner				
	Bedtime				

Notes :

Date	Meal	Time	Before	After	Med/Insulin
THU	Breakfast				
	Lunch				
	Dinner				
	Bedtime				

Notes :

Date	Meal	Time	Before	After	Med/Insulin
FRI	Breakfast				
	Lunch				
	Dinner				
	Bedtime				

Notes :

Date	Meal	Time	Before	After	Med/Insulin
SAT	Breakfast				
	Lunch				
	Dinner				
	Bedtime				

Notes :

Date	Meal	Time	Before	After	Med/Insulin
SUN	Breakfast				
	Lunch				
	Dinner				
	Bedtime				

Notes :

Notes :

Week :					Weight :	
Date	Meal	Time	Before	After	Med/Insulin	
MON	Breakfast					
	Lunch					
	Dinner					
	Bedtime					

Notes :

Date	Meal	Time	Before	After	Med/Insulin	
TUE	Breakfast					
	Lunch					
	Dinner					
	Bedtime					

Notes :

Date	Meal	Time	Before	After	Med/Insulin	
WED	Breakfast					
	Lunch					
	Dinner					
	Bedtime					

Notes :

Date	Meal	Time	Before	After	Med/Insulin	
THU	Breakfast					
	Lunch					
	Dinner					
	Bedtime					

Notes :

Date	Meal	Time	Before	After	Med/Insulin
FRI	Breakfast				
	Lunch				
	Dinner				
	Bedtime				

Notes :

Date	Meal	Time	Before	After	Med/Insulin
SAT	Breakfast				
	Lunch				
	Dinner				
	Bedtime				

Notes :

Date	Meal	Time	Before	After	Med/Insulin
SUN	Breakfast				
	Lunch				
	Dinner				
	Bedtime				

Notes :

Notes :

Week :				Weight :	
Date	Meal	Time	Before	After	Med/Insulin
MON	Breakfast				
	Lunch				
	Dinner				
	Bedtime				
Notes :					

Date	Meal	Time	Before	After	Med/Insulin
TUE	Breakfast				
	Lunch				
	Dinner				
	Bedtime				
Notes :					

Date	Meal	Time	Before	After	Med/Insulin
WED	Breakfast				
	Lunch				
	Dinner				
	Bedtime				
Notes :					

Date	Meal	Time	Before	After	Med/Insulin
THU	Breakfast				
	Lunch				
	Dinner				
	Bedtime				
Notes :					

Date	Meal	Time	Before	After	Med/Insulin
FRI	Breakfast				
	Lunch				
	Dinner				
	Bedtime				

Notes :

Date	Meal	Time	Before	After	Med/Insulin
SAT	Breakfast				
	Lunch				
	Dinner				
	Bedtime				

Notes :

Date	Meal	Time	Before	After	Med/Insulin
SUN	Breakfast				
	Lunch				
	Dinner				
	Bedtime				

Notes :

Notes :

Week :				Weight :	

Date	Meal	Time	Before	After	Med/Insulin
MON	Breakfast				
	Lunch				
	Dinner				
	Bedtime				

Notes :

Date	Meal	Time	Before	After	Med/Insulin
TUE	Breakfast				
	Lunch				
	Dinner				
	Bedtime				

Notes :

Date	Meal	Time	Before	After	Med/Insulin
WED	Breakfast				
	Lunch				
	Dinner				
	Bedtime				

Notes :

Date	Meal	Time	Before	After	Med/Insulin
THU	Breakfast				
	Lunch				
	Dinner				
	Bedtime				

Notes :

Date	Meal	Time	Before	After	Med/Insulin
FRI	Breakfast				
	Lunch				
	Dinner				
	Bedtime				

Notes :

Date	Meal	Time	Before	After	Med/Insulin
SAT	Breakfast				
	Lunch				
	Dinner				
	Bedtime				

Notes :

Date	Meal	Time	Before	After	Med/Insulin
SUN	Breakfast				
	Lunch				
	Dinner				
	Bedtime				

Notes :

Notes :

Week :				Weight :	
Date	Meal	Time	Before	After	Med/Insulin
MON	Breakfast				
	Lunch				
	Dinner				
	Bedtime				

Notes :

Date	Meal	Time	Before	After	Med/Insulin
TUE	Breakfast				
	Lunch				
	Dinner				
	Bedtime				

Notes :

Date	Meal	Time	Before	After	Med/Insulin
WED	Breakfast				
	Lunch				
	Dinner				
	Bedtime				

Notes :

Date	Meal	Time	Before	After	Med/Insulin
THU	Breakfast				
	Lunch				
	Dinner				
	Bedtime				

Notes :

Date	Meal	Time	Before	After	Med/Insulin
FRI	Breakfast				
	Lunch				
	Dinner				
	Bedtime				
Notes :					

Date	Meal	Time	Before	After	Med/Insulin
SAT	Breakfast				
	Lunch				
	Dinner				
	Bedtime				
Notes :					

Date	Meal	Time	Before	After	Med/Insulin
SUN	Breakfast				
	Lunch				
	Dinner				
	Bedtime				
Notes :					

Notes :

Week :				Weight :	

Date	Meal	Time	Before	After	Med/Insulin
MON	Breakfast				
	Lunch				
	Dinner				
	Bedtime				

Notes :

Date	Meal	Time	Before	After	Med/Insulin
TUE	Breakfast				
	Lunch				
	Dinner				
	Bedtime				

Notes :

Date	Meal	Time	Before	After	Med/Insulin
WED	Breakfast				
	Lunch				
	Dinner				
	Bedtime				

Notes :

Date	Meal	Time	Before	After	Med/Insulin
THU	Breakfast				
	Lunch				
	Dinner				
	Bedtime				

Notes :

Date	Meal	Time	Before	After	Med/Insulin
FRI	Breakfast				
	Lunch				
	Dinner				
	Bedtime				

Notes :

Date	Meal	Time	Before	After	Med/Insulin
SAT	Breakfast				
	Lunch				
	Dinner				
	Bedtime				

Notes :

Date	Meal	Time	Before	After	Med/Insulin
SUN	Breakfast				
	Lunch				
	Dinner				
	Bedtime				

Notes :

Notes :

Week :				Weight :	

Date	Meal	Time	Before	After	Med/Insulin
MON	Breakfast				
	Lunch				
	Dinner				
	Bedtime				

Notes :

Date	Meal	Time	Before	After	Med/Insulin
TUE	Breakfast				
	Lunch				
	Dinner				
	Bedtime				

Notes :

Date	Meal	Time	Before	After	Med/Insulin
WED	Breakfast				
	Lunch				
	Dinner				
	Bedtime				

Notes :

Date	Meal	Time	Before	After	Med/Insulin
THU	Breakfast				
	Lunch				
	Dinner				
	Bedtime				

Notes :

Date	Meal	Time	Before	After	Med/Insulin
FRI	Breakfast				
	Lunch				
	Dinner				
	Bedtime				

Notes :

Date	Meal	Time	Before	After	Med/Insulin
SAT	Breakfast				
	Lunch				
	Dinner				
	Bedtime				

Notes :

Date	Meal	Time	Before	After	Med/Insulin
SUN	Breakfast				
	Lunch				
	Dinner				
	Bedtime				

Notes :

Notes :

Week :				Weight :	

Date	Meal	Time	Before	After	Med/Insulin
MON	Breakfast				
	Lunch				
	Dinner				
	Bedtime				

Notes :

Date	Meal	Time	Before	After	Med/Insulin
TUE	Breakfast				
	Lunch				
	Dinner				
	Bedtime				

Notes :

Date	Meal	Time	Before	After	Med/Insulin
WED	Breakfast				
	Lunch				
	Dinner				
	Bedtime				

Notes :

Date	Meal	Time	Before	After	Med/Insulin
THU	Breakfast				
	Lunch				
	Dinner				
	Bedtime				

Notes :

Date	Meal	Time	Before	After	Med/Insulin
FRI	Breakfast				
	Lunch				
	Dinner				
	Bedtime				

Notes :

Date	Meal	Time	Before	After	Med/Insulin
SAT	Breakfast				
	Lunch				
	Dinner				
	Bedtime				

Notes :

Date	Meal	Time	Before	After	Med/Insulin
SUN	Breakfast				
	Lunch				
	Dinner				
	Bedtime				

Notes :

Notes :

- -

- -

- -

- -

- -

- -

- -

- -

Week :				Weight :	
Date	Meal	Time	Before	After	Med/Insulin
MON	Breakfast				
	Lunch				
	Dinner				
	Bedtime				

Notes :

Date	Meal	Time	Before	After	Med/Insulin
TUE	Breakfast				
	Lunch				
	Dinner				
	Bedtime				

Notes :

Date	Meal	Time	Before	After	Med/Insulin
WED	Breakfast				
	Lunch				
	Dinner				
	Bedtime				

Notes :

Date	Meal	Time	Before	After	Med/Insulin
THU	Breakfast				
	Lunch				
	Dinner				
	Bedtime				

Notes :

Date	Meal	Time	Before	After	Med/Insulin
FRI	Breakfast				
	Lunch				
	Dinner				
	Bedtime				

Notes :

Date	Meal	Time	Before	After	Med/Insulin
SAT	Breakfast				
	Lunch				
	Dinner				
	Bedtime				

Notes :

Date	Meal	Time	Before	After	Med/Insulin
SUN	Breakfast				
	Lunch				
	Dinner				
	Bedtime				

Notes :

Notes :

Week :				Weight :	
Date	Meal	Time	Before	After	Med/Insulin
MON	Breakfast				
	Lunch				
	Dinner				
	Bedtime				

Notes :

Date	Meal	Time	Before	After	Med/Insulin
TUE	Breakfast				
	Lunch				
	Dinner				
	Bedtime				

Notes :

Date	Meal	Time	Before	After	Med/Insulin
WED	Breakfast				
	Lunch				
	Dinner				
	Bedtime				

Notes :

Date	Meal	Time	Before	After	Med/Insulin
THU	Breakfast				
	Lunch				
	Dinner				
	Bedtime				

Notes :

Date	Meal	Time	Before	After	Med/Insulin
FRI	Breakfast				
	Lunch				
	Dinner				
	Bedtime				

Notes :

Date	Meal	Time	Before	After	Med/Insulin
SAT	Breakfast				
	Lunch				
	Dinner				
	Bedtime				

Notes :

Date	Meal	Time	Before	After	Med/Insulin
SUN	Breakfast				
	Lunch				
	Dinner				
	Bedtime				

Notes :

Notes :

NOTES

NOTES

NOTES

NOTES

NOTES

THANK YOU FOR PURCHASING THIS BOOK

WITHOUT YOUR VOICE WE WOULD BE LOST.
HELP US MAKE BETTER BOOKS BY LEAVING
AN HONEST REVIEW ON
AMAZON

SCAN YOUR COUNTRY QR CODE
TO BUY THIS BOOK
OR
LEAVE AN HONEST REVIEW

USA

UK

CA

Made in United States
North Haven, CT
24 March 2024